MRCPsych Part 1
Practice Questions

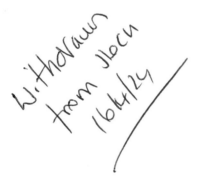

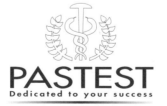

PASTEST
Dedicated to your success

MRCPsych Part 1
Practice Questions

Gin S. Malhi
MBChB, BSc (Hons), MRCPsych, FRANCP
School of Psychiatry, University of New South Wales,
Sydney, Australia

Bob S. Malhi
MBBS, MRCPsych
Charing Cross and Westminster Hospitals, London, UK

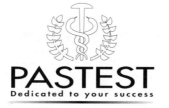

PASTEST
Dedicated to your success

First published 2004

ISBN: 1 901198 01 3

A catalogue record for this book is available from the British Library.

The information contained within this book was obtained by the authors from reliable sources. However, while every effort has been made to ensure its accuracy, no responsibility for loss, damage or injury occasioned to any person acting or refraining from action as a result of information contained herein can be accepted by the publishers or authors.

PasTest Revision Books and Intensive Courses

PasTest has been established in the field of postgraduate medical education since 1972, providing revision books and intensive study courses for doctors preparing for their professional examinations.

Books and courses are available for the following specialties:
MRCGP, MRCP Part 1 and 2, MRCPCH Part 1 and 2, MRCPsych, MRCS, MRCOG, DRCOG, DCH, FRCA, PLAB.

For further details contact:

PasTest, Freepost, Knutsford, Cheshire WA16 7BR
Tel: 01565 752000   Fax: 01565 650264
www.pastest.co.uk   enquiries@pastest.co.uk

Cover design by Old Tin Dog Design Company
Text prepared by Saxon Graphics Ltd, Derby
Printed and bound by Page Bros (Norwich Ltd)

Contents

Preface

The MRCPsych examination is administered by the Royal College of Psychiatrists twice a year and consists of two parts. This book is written for the Part 1 written examination paper which is made up of a combination of individual statement questions (ISQs), which are either true or false, and extended matching items (EMIs) questions, in which the answer is selected from a list of choices.

The curriculum is covered in the ten chapters of this book. Each chapter focuses on a single subject area, such as basic psychology, psychopharmacology or psychotherapy.

Preparation for the examination should begin in good time and most candidates require a period of four to six months. It is important from the outset to be equipped with the appropriate texts and have a clear idea of the format of the examination and the extent of knowledge required. It is best therefore to obtain, from the Royal College, the latest guidelines in place at the time of application.

Revision should be tailored to the examination and ideally a set time should be put aside on a daily basis. Questions can be used to revise new learning and test knowledge but it is essential to attempt a complete paper under examination conditions.

Even with the best preparation there is bound to be some anxiety both in the days before the examination and on the day itself. Ideally, this should be used to focus learning and enhance performance but this too requires practice.

This book has been written with these considerations in mind and it is hoped that it will be of help to those sitting the MRCPsych Part 1 Examination.

To help you revise for your objective structured clinical examination (OSCE), read *OSCEs for MRCPsych Part 1*, also published by PasTest, ISBN 1 904627 04 8.

G S Mahli
B S Malhi

Foreword

A career in hospital medicine is a series of journeys, from life as a student to that of a Consultant. All journeys have a beginning and an end. For a psychiatrist, the journey starts with an attraction to the field of mental illness, where one comes face to face with the vulnerabilities of their highly evolved brain. There are many facts to learn, many skills to acquire and many patients to see. Basic specialist training is followed by higher specialist training and then life-long continuing professional development.

Progress through basic specialist training is marked by passing the examinations of the Royal College of Psychiatrists for which there is a daunting curriculum to master. At first glance it may seem that there is no limit to the depth of knowledge that is required. The curriculum is at the same time broad in parts, narrow in others, detailed on one page and vague on the next.

Time is a precious commodity for the working doctor who must revise effectively for the examinations. It is of little surprise then that a wide range of revision books have been published over the years. However, the Examinations Sub-Committee of the Royal College of Psychiatrists has not stood still. It adapts the examinations regularly to the training needs of psychiatrists and old methods of assessment are superseded by modern ones. The changes have been particularly dramatic over the last few years as the pace of educational reform has quickened.

It is welcome news then that PasTest, the leading provider of medical revision courses and books, now enters the field of psychiatric education. Using experienced authors, it introduces a brand new range of up-to-date revision books for trainee psychiatrists, of which this book is the first.

Malhi and Malhi have written this book for those doctors taking the MRCPsych Part I examination, the first major hurdle in the journey of trainee psychiatrists. The examination consists of two parts, a written paper followed by the objective structured clinical examination

(OSCE). This book helps doctors prepare for the written paper which is made up of a combination of individual statement questions (ISQs), which are either true or false, and extended matching items (EMIs) questions, in which the answer is selected from a list of choices.

The abolition of negative marking, where wrong answers lose marks, means that candidates should attempt all questions. Candidates can only sit the OSCE if they score a satisfactory mark in the written paper. In recent examinations, 55–60% of candidates passed the written paper which is criterion referenced marked, that is, the pass mark which identifies a sufficiently prepared candidate is decided by the Examination Sub-Committee and every candidate who achieves that mark passes the examination. This is in contrast to the older peer referenced marking that used to be employed in the College examinations, where only a certain percentage of the candidates passed, regardless of the ability of the whole cohort.

Even a cursory glance through this book will send shivers down the spines of experienced psychiatrists, for the questions mirror those found in the real examination. That is a good thing, for there is nothing worse than practising answering questions that bear little resemblance to the real ones. The standard of difficulty of the questions in this book is exactly right.

The curriculum is covered in its entirety in the ten chapters of this book. Each chapter focuses on a single area of the curriculum, such as basic psychology, psychopharmacology or psychotherapy. This aids the revision process, for the reader can learn in stages and by answering the questions chapter by chapter, identify the weakest areas of his or her knowledge. Using the book regularly will help the reader to accurately judge the breadth and depth of knowledge required to pass the exam. A revision strategy that balances knowledge across all areas of the curriculum is sensible. Areas that are neglected are always examined on!

Of course questions are no good without answers and this book includes explanatory answers for all the questions, even for those statements which are true. The answers are written using concise, clear language and perhaps uniquely for a psychiatric book, there is no sense of ambiguity.

Malhi and Malhi are to be congratulated on writing an excellent book. It deserves to sit on the bookshelves of all trainee psychiatrists who will be richly rewarded for using it in their exam preparation. The journey may be difficult but at least now it is better lit.

Gurpal Singh Gosall MA MB BChir MRCPsych
Specialist Registrar, General Adult Psychiatry
Manchester

Chapter 1: Basic Psychology

1.1
In associative learning, the optimum delay between the uncon-ditioned stimulus and the conditioned stimulus is 0.5 seconds.

1.2
The time to acquire an association in classical conditioning is known as the procurement stage.

1.3
In operant conditioning, a variable schedule of reinforcement is more effective at maintaining a desired behaviour than contingency reinforcement.

1.4
Reciprocal inhibition is based on the ideas of Wolpe.

1.5
Negative reinforcement is achieved by the administration of an aversive stimulus in response to an unwanted behaviour.

1.6
Watson and Rayner demonstrated phobia generalisation.

1.7
If classical conditioning is successful the unconditioned response becomes the conditioned stimulus.

1.8
Classical conditioning is also known as respondent learning.

1.9
Vicarious learning is associated with Bandura.

1.10
Size constancy is important in Gestalt principles of perception.

1.11
Object constancy is an alternative term for object permanence.

1.12
A perceptual set influences the way something is perceived.

1.13
In describing conditions for optimal observational learning, Bandura used perceptual theory.

1.14
The id is wholly unconscious.

1.15
The Yerkes–Dodson curve plots performance against level of arousal.

1.16
Chaining and shaping are ways of achieving a desired behaviour based on operant techniques.

1.17
The 'need for achievement' described by McClelland is an emotional model of motivation.

1.18
Seligman's notion of learned helplessness forms part of the psychological model of depression.

1.19
In perception the whole is very often greater than the sum of its parts.

1.20
The Weber–Fechner law relates stimulus intensity to how strongly it is perceived.

Chapter 2: Neuropsychological Assessment

2.1
The 'draw a person test' is a projective personality test.

2.2
The National Adult Reading Test (NART) is used as a measure of pre-morbid IQ.

2.3
In relation to data collection, the leniency error is explained by a positive rapport between the subject and the interviewer.

2.4
Thalamic processing is central to the James-Lange theory of emotion.

2.5
Festinger's cognitive dissonance theory can be considered a theory of motivation.

2.6
Nomothetic research derives information from studying individuals.

2.7
In Maslow's hierarchy of needs, understanding comes before aesthetic concerns.

2.8
The validity of a test is the extent to which it generates consistent results on repeated administration at different times or by different researchers.

2.9
There is no such thing as 'global intelligence'.

2.10
Kretschmer described endomorphs as people who sought enjoyment and relaxation.

2.11
Digit span and digit symbol are both part of the WAIS-III-R.

2.12
The WAIS-III-R is often incorporated into the Halsted–Reitan Neuropsychological Battery (HRNB).

2.13
In his trait theory of personality, Cattel used factor analysis to derive 16 first-order personality factors.

2.14
The primacy and recency effects explain enhancements in immediate memory on the basis of the order in which data is presented.

2.15
Secondary memory can be divided into declarative and procedural aspects.

2.16
The Thurstone scale consists of ranked statements from which subjects choose those they agree with.

2.17
Social responses are a naturally occurring reinforcer of behaviour.

2.18
Prosody is usually controlled by the left temporal lobe.

2.19
The majority of left-handed individuals show left hemisphere dominance of speech.

2.20
Olfactory sensation is the only sense to be projected mainly to the ipsilateral hemisphere.

Chapter 3: Human Growth and Development

3.1
In Piaget's model of cognitive development novel stimuli are assimilated into existing schemas.

3.2
Concerning Kleinian theory, the depressive position is linked to manic defences.

3.3
Piaget's model pertains principally to cognitive development.

3.4
In Kleinian theory, the paranoid-schizoid position develops in the first year of life.

3.5
The latent period in Freud's theory of development begins post-puberty.

3.6
Freud's theory of development pertains principally to emotional development.

3.7
Karl Abraham, a student of Freud's, further subdivided the phallic phase of Freud's psychosexual theory.

3.8
In Freud's oral stage infants show ambivalence towards objects.

3.9
In Margaret Mahler's theory of development, the autistic phase occurs in the infant's second year.

3.10
In Margaret Mahler's theory of development, there are four subphases of separation–individuation.

3.11
According to Freud's psychosexual theory the ego develops during the anal stage.

3.12
In the Electra complex as described by Freud, the girl believes she once had a penis which has since been removed.

3.13
In Freud's theory of development, identification with the same-sex parent heralds the end of the phallic phase.

3.14
In Erikson's oral–sensory stage, the main crisis centres around trust–mistrust.

3.15
The psychosocial moratorium pertains to the stage between latency and adolescence in Erikson's theory.

3.16
The central theme in Erikson's final stage of development is integrity versus despair.

3.17
In Freud's theory of development, mimicry of the same-sex parent occurs in the latent phase.

3.18
Margaret Mahler used the empirical method to develop her ideas.

3.19
Erikson was the first classical development theorist to develop a comprehensive lifelong scheme.

3.20
Separation from the caregiver at 2 months usually distresses the child.

3.21
Thomas and Chess categorised three main types of child temperament.

3.22
Monotropic attachment is usually established by 6 months.

3.23
In Piaget's model of cognitive development, object permanence first appears at around 2 years.

3.24
Kohlberg's theory of moral development was based on the responses of subjects presented with stories posing moral dilemmas.

3.25
Some individuals may never reach the level of post-conventional morality described in Kohlberg's theory of moral development.

3.26
Lorenz explained attachment as a form of imprinting.

3.27
Babies are born with a fixed visual focus of 1 metre.

3.28
6:6 visual acuity is acquired by 6 months of age.

3.29
By 2 years, most children have a vocabulary of 500 words.

3.30
Language is slower to develop in children with no siblings.

3.31
Stimulus preparedness involves being forewarned of a potential fear-provoking stimulus.

3.32
Gender role refers to a person's self-awareness as a male or female.

3.33
Gender identity is usually achieved by 3 years.

3.34
Thelarche is usually the first sign of puberty in girls.

3.35
Grief typically resolves within 6 months, after which it may be an atypical reaction.

3.36
Kübler-Ross described five phases of adjustment on being confronted with the knowledge of one's own imminent death.

3.37
Memory inevitably declines with age.

3.38
Intelligence generally increases up until middle-age.

3.39
There is an increased incidence of homosexuality in those who have been sexually abused as children compared with those who have not.

3.40
Children who have been physically abused themselves are less likely to later abuse their own children.

Chapter 4: Psychopathology

4.1
Écho de la pensée is a Schneiderian first-rank symptom.

4.2
Logoclonia is a form of perseveration.

4.3
Asyndesis is a term for 'loosening of association' of thought.

4.4
Alexithymia is the inability to control one's emotions adequately.

4.5
Vorbeigehen describes a tendency to give incorrect or approximate answers that nevertheless reveal the question has been understood.

4.6
Entgleisen is another term for thought block.

4.7
An apophanous perception is a Schneiderian first-rank symptom.

4.8
Capgras syndrome comprises nihilistic delusions.

4.9
Catatonia and stupor are equivalent terms.

4.10
Gedankenlautwerden is a Schneiderian symptom.

4.11
Pressure of thought and pressure of speech essentially allude to the same phenomenon.

4.12
Delusions are invariably false.

4.13
Informal thought disorder is a milder subtype of thought disorder which is not commonly used.

4.14
Thought echo is a disorder of thought possession.

4.15
Reflex hallucinations are a synaesthetic phenomenon.

4.16
Pareidolic illusions can occur in healthy individuals.

4.17
A delusional perception can often be understood with reference to the individual's mental state.

4.18
Hallucinations can occur in healthy people.

4.19
Delusions may occur in healthy people.

4.20
Passivity phenomena are sometimes referred to as delusions of control.

4.21
Alexithymia is an inability to express one's emotions.

4.22
An individual with Fregoli syndrome is likely to be over-familiar with a stranger.

4.23
'Affect' is said to be a more short-term reflection of one's emotions than 'mood'.

4.24
In the context of a mental state examination, 'incongruity' describes antisocial or challenging behaviour.

4.25
In functional hallucinations, a (correct) percept produces a distinct hallucination in the same modality.

4.26
Lilliputian hallucinations are often associated with pleasure.

4.27
Strictly speaking, ruminations are an example of thought insertion.

4.28
Prolixity is a less severe form of flight of ideas in which the goal of thought is eventually reached.

4.29
Dysmorphophobia can be treated surgically.

4.30
Topographic amnesia is well recognised in Alzheimer's disease.

4.31
Concerning passivity phenomena, the affected individual does not always attribute the experience to an outside agency.

4.32
Witzelsucht: apathy and silliness combined with general indifference.

4.33
Paralogia is the verbal expression of positive thought disorder.

4.34
Delusions of misidentification include reduplicative paramnesia.

4.35
Akinesis is a term for flight of ideas.

4.36
Primary delusions only occur in functional psychoses.

4.37
Neologisms are characteristic of formal thought disorder.

4.38
Parsimony is often associated with personality.

4.39
Couvade's syndrome and pseudocyesis are synonymous.

4.40
De Claramboult's syndrome is a psychotic disorder.

4.41
An autochthonous delusion is synonymous with *Wahreinfall*.

4.42
A negative hallucination is so termed because it causes intense fear.

4.43
An apophanous delusion is a form of primary delusion.

4.44
Haptic hallucinations are recognised in cocaine use.

4.45
Extracampine hallucinations are visual.

4.46
Autoscopy is a variety of auditory hallucination in which the patient hears their own voice.

4.47
Patients often consider their overvalued ideas to be senseless.

4.48
Partial delusions are equivalent to overvalued ideas.

4.49
Vertigo can be described as an hallucination of the vestibular system.

4.50
Simple auditory hallucinations are so-called because they are easy for the patient to understand.

4.51
Wahnstimmung characteristically precedes the onset of delusional thinking.

4.52
Mimicry of speech is also referred to as verbigeration.

4.53
Delusional memories occur in those recovering from delusional experiences.

4.54
Jamais vu describes the experience of never having seen a familiar sight before.

4.55
In parakinesia the patient approximately mimics another's movements.

4.56
Negativism is characteristic of depression.

4.57
Lilliputian hallucinations are a form of micropsia.

4.58
In thought broadcasting the essential experience is of one's thoughts being transmitted from the mind.

4.59
Formication is associated with delirious states.

4.60
Hypochondriacal delusions are always false.

4.61
The content of confabulation is usually false.

4.62
Second-person auditory hallucinations are so called because they involve the simultaneous perception of more than one voice.

4.63
Autoscopic hallucinations do not occur in healthy people.

4.64
Depersonalisation involves a change in the subjective experience of one's self such that one feels unreal or detached from reality.

4.65
The 'psychological pillow' is a term used by psychologists to describe a comfort zone for the patient.

4.66
Ambitendency describes the phenomenon of wanting to use both hands to perform a one-handed task.

4.67
In reduplicative phenomena the patient believes parts of the body, or the whole body, have been duplicated.

4.68
Phantom limb is the lay term for hemisomatognosia.

4.69
Coenestopathic states are a form of body image disorder.

4.70
Mitgehen is automatic obedience.

4.71
In palinacousis there is perseveration of an auditory percept.

4.72
Hygric hallucinations involve the perception of heat.

4.73
Stereotypical movements lack any obvious function.

4.74
In the oneiroid state a person experiences dream-like imagery but is not asleep.

4.75
The Omega sign is characteristically seen in depression.

4.76
Autoscopic hallucinations can sometimes give rise to a *Doppelgänger*.

4.77
Torpor is a term for neuroleptic-induced bradykinesia

4.78
Schnauzkrampf is seen in catatonic schizophrenia.

4.79
Cataplexy describes a trance-like state with loss of voluntary movement.

4.80
Subjects with an eidetic memory experience recalled information as a visual pseudohallucination.

Chapter 5: Psychopharmacology

5.1
Primidone, a precursor of phenobarbitone, is teratogenic.

5.2
Norfluoxetine, a metabolite of fluoxetine, is eliminated by the kidneys.

5.3
Fluoxetine has a half-life of one week.

5.4
Ethosuximide is secreted in breast milk.

5.5
Iodine is secreted in breast milk.

5.6
Moclobemide, a reversible inhibitor of monoamine oxidase A (RIMA), can be used in the treatment of social phobia.

5.7
Lithium usually causes heightened T-waves on an ECG.

5.8
Chlordiazepoxide is absorbed unchanged from the gastrointestinal tract.

5.9
Sodium valproate administration in the first trimester of pregnancy increases the risk of neural-tube defects.

5.10
In those with moral disorders taking Lithium the concurrent use of acetazolamide increases the risk of relapse.

5.11
Lithium accentuates physiological tremor.

5.12
Benzodiazepines suppress EEG activity across the range of measured frequencies.

5.13
Disulfiram decreases plasma levels of chlordiazepoxide.

5.14
Chronic phenytoin use can lead to megaloblastic anaemia.

5.15
Aripipazola is a partial D_2 agonist.

5.16
Phenobarbitone can impair infant breast-feeding.

5.17
Pericyazine is an atypical antipsychotic.

5.18
Methixene is an anticholinergic drug used in Parkinsonism.

5.19
Cardiac failure impairs intramuscular absorption of drugs.

5.20
Chronic lithium administration decreases serotonergic neurotransmission.

5.21
Anticholinesterases inhibit the progression of dementia, but only for as long as the patient continues to take them.

5.22
CNS serotonin is metabolised mainly by MAO-B.

5.23
Chronic lithium treatment increases erythrocyte choline levels.

5.24
Lithium treatment can decrease central dopamine synthesis.

5.25
Long-term chlorpromazine administration may cause opacity of the lens.

5.26
Pyrexia is a recognised side-effect of clozapine.

5.27
Agranulocytosis is a recognised dose-dependent side-effect of neuroleptics.

5.28
Tinnitus is associated with lithium intoxication.

5.29
Long-term lithium treatment causes arrhythmias and memory impairment.

5.30
Testicular enlargement is a recognised side-effect of tricyclic anti-depressants.

5.31
Carbamazepine can cause ataxia at therapeutic doses.

5.32
Phenelzine is not sedative.

5.33
The combination of tranylcypromine and clomipramine is safer than most other combinations of these two classes of drug.

5.34
Propranolol may be used to potentiate antidepressants.

5.35
Sodium valproate is associated with weight gain.

5.36
Smoking has been shown to reduce plasma levels of olemzapine.

5.37
Propranolol, neuroleptics and TCAs may all cause erectile failure.

5.38
Lithium exacerbates psoriasis.

5.39
Diuresis is a recognised side-effect of carbamazepine.

5.40
Carbamazepine can be used safely in combination with phenelzine.

5.41
Pancytopenia is a recognised side-effect of carbamazepine.

5.42
Sulpiride should be avoided in pregnancy but is safe in breast-feeding.

5.43
TCAs can cause galactorrhoea.

5.44
Ranitidine has been associated with a toxic confusional psychosis.

5.45
TCAs enhance MAOI action.

5.46
Benzhexol is more sedating than benztropine.

5.47
Depression is a recognised side-effect of clonidine.

5.48
Dothiepin is more sedating than lofepramine.

5.49
L-Tryptophan can be used to treat insomnia.

5.50
L-Dopa is metabolised in the brain.

5.51
Alcohol and phenytoin metabolism observes first-order kinetics.

5.52
Dopamine antagonists can cause retinitis.

5.53
Tardive dyskinesia is as troubling for relatives as for the affected individual.

5.54
Fresh fish is safe for those taking isocarboxacid.

5.55
Chlorpromazine and amitriptyline increase $\propto$ and θ activity on an EEG.

5.56
Lithium does not significantly alter EEG recordings.

5.57
L-Tryptophan is an important neurotransmitter in the mediation of depression.

5.58
Domperidone is a dopamine antagonist.

5.59
Visual hallucinations occur with anticholinergic toxicity.

5.60
Der sensitive Beziehungswahn describes a personality predisposed to persecutory delusions.

5.61
Dopamine is implicated in the monoamine hypothesis of depression.

5.62
α-Methyl-para-tyrosine (AMPT) can precipitate depression in healthy subjects.

5.63
Maprotilene is a tetracyclic antidepressant that inhibits serotonin reuptake.

5.64
The steady state of a drug is usually achieved in three half-lives.

5.65
A QTc interval of more than 450 mg is of potential concern.

5.66
Peak lithium concentrations are usually achieved in around six hours.

5.67
Regarding pregnant women taking lithium, Ebstein's anomaly is seen in 1% of births.

5.68
Sodium valproate use is associated with hirsuitism in women.

5.69
Carbamazepine is considered to be of value in the management of aggression.

5.70
Topiramate usually causes weight gain.

5.71
Gabapentin has a narrow therapeutic index (TI).

5.72
Tolerance to benzodiazepines does not usually develop before four weeks of continuous use.

5.73
Benzodiazepines typically reduce REM sleep in the initial stages of treatment before tolerance develops.

5.74
Buspirone has been shown to be effective in panic disorder.

5.75
Tardive dyskinesia is an entirely iatrogenic condition.

5.76
Tardive dyskinesia generally affects women more than men.

5.77
Clozapine and amilsulpiride are both beneficial in the treatment of negative symptoms of schizophrenia.

5.78
Long-term NSAIDs increase the risk of Alzheimer's disease.

5.79
Donepezil potentiates suxamethonium.

5.80
Atypical neuroleptics have so far not been implicated in cases of neuroleptic malignant syndrome (NMS).

Chapter 6: Psychiatric Disorders

6.1
Balloon cells are a characteristic feature of Pick's disease.

6.2
Corpus callosum thinning is seen in dementia pugilistica.

6.3
Ventricular enlargement is more common in multi-infarct dementia than in Alzheimer's disease.

6.4
Presenelin-2 on chromosome 14 is found in approximately 75% of early-onset familial Alzheimer's disease.

6.5
Schizophreniform psychosis is a recognised association of Parkinson's disease.

6.6
Retrograde amnesia is a characteristic feature of Korsakoff's psychosis.

6.7
Following a head injury dementia does not occur provided the skull is intact.

6.8
Constructional dyspraxia is more commonly seen in organic dementias than in a depressive pseudodementia.

6.9
Mild euphoria is more commonly seen than anger in the prodromal phase of an epileptic seizure.

6.10

Organic cerebral dysfunction is suspected when there is a discrepancy of 10 or more between the verbal and performance scores on the WAIS-R.

6.11

Echopraxia and echolalia are both seen in Tourette's syndrome.

6.12

The EEG in Alzheimer's disease shows focal δ-wave activity.

6.13

In schizophrenia, life events are more significant in terms of the course of illness and risk of relapse rather than its onset.

6.14

The lifetime risk of a child developing schizophrenia is doubled if both parents are affected rather than just one.

6.15

Ekbom's syndrome involves delusions of infestation.

6.16

The incidence of homicidal behaviour in schizophrenia is around 10%.

6.17

Delusional mood is a characteristic feature of psychotic depression.

6.18

Good prognostic indicators in schizophrenia include an abrupt onset.

6.19

Following a closed head injury, the incidence of new-onset epilepsy is 5–10%.

6.20

In post-ictal psychoses, delusions occur more commonly than in schizophrenia.

6.21
The so-called 'winter births' bias seen in schizophrenia spans October to February.

6.22
Morbid jealousy is reduced by the proximity of the partner.

6.23
Pain of psychological origin tends to worsen with time.

6.24
Schizophrenia is associated with HLA 2C.

6.25
Concerning the fathers of individuals with schizophrenia, a higher proportion stems from social class V than class I.

6.26
Biological families of schizophrenia show an increased prevalence of alcohol problems.

6.27
Violence in schizophrenia is related to premorbid psychosocial functioning.

6.28
Schneiderian first-rank symptoms in schizophrenia are useful prognostic indicators.

6.29
Schneiderian first-rank symptoms are not present in approximately half of all diagnosed cases of schizophrenia.

6.30
Unusual or embarrassing sexual behaviour is seen in around 25% of those with chronic schizophrenia.

6.31
Schizoid traits are not relevant in the prognosis of schizophrenia.

6.32
Dysplasia of the medial temporal lobes occurs in schizophrenia.

6.33
Unipolar depressive disorders are equally common in both sexes.

6.34
There is an increased risk of bipolar illness in the first-degree relatives of a subject with unipolar illness.

6.35
The typical age of onset of unipolar illness is generally a decade earlier than in bipolar illness.

6.36
In depression, stages 3 and 4 of sleep are decreased.

6.37
Mannerisms are a common feature of mania.

6.38
Morbid jealousy generally carries a good prognosis.

6.39
Histrionic behaviour is a recognised feature of depression.

6.40
Carbohydrate cravings are typical of seasonal affective disorder.

6.41
Transient periods of depressed mood are characteristic of a hypomanic state.

6.42
In severe depression there can be an absence of sadness.

6.43
Affective psychosis disorders are more frequent following head injury than schizophrenic psychosis.

6.44
Around 20% of depressive episodes require inpatient treatment.

6.45
The distinction between hypomania and mania is based on strict operational criteria, that are clinically meaningful.

6.46
Patients with recurrent brief depressive disorder are depressed most of the time.

6.47
Melancholia is characterised by psychomotor retardation.

6.48
A diagnosis of rapid cycling disorder is conventionally made on the basis of at least three distinct episodes of affective illness (each sufficient to meet diagnostic criteria) in one year.

6.49
Genetic influences appear to be greater in bipolar than unipolar disorders.

6.50
Bereavement can precipitate mania.

6.51
A family history of mental illness is often present in puerperal psychosis.

6.52
Ambivalence toward the pregnancy is an important risk factor for puerperal psychosis.

6.53
Neurotic disorders are rarely seen in the over-65s.

6.54
Agoraphobia is worse on a train than in a car.

6.55
Depersonalisation is associated with phobic anxiety.

6.56
Fugue is a recognised complication of severe depression.

6.57
Dysmorphophobia can remit after surgery.

6.58
Depersonalisation is not often seen in obsessional disorders.

6.59
Agoraphobia has a mean age of onset in the third decade of life.

6.60
Neurotic disability is the commonest psychiatric sequel to head injury.

6.61
The alternative personalities seen in multiple personality disorder are most commonly those of children.

6.62
Symptoms of post-traumatic stress disorder are more likely following natural rather than man-made disasters.

6.63
Astasia–abasia is regarded as a dissociative state.

6.64
Depersonalisation is often associated with a change in mood.

6.65
Hypochondriasis is a delusional disorder.

6.66
Obsessive rituals can increase anxiety.

6.67
There is strong evidence of twin-pair concordance in conversion disorders.

6.68
Primary amenorrhoea is a recognised feature of generalised anxiety disorder.

6.69
Panic attacks are less often a feature of agoraphobia than of other phobic disorders.

6.70
Hypochondriacal delusions are seen in hypochondriasis.

6.71
Vertigo is a characteristic symptom of acute anxiety.

6.72
Agoraphobic symptoms tend not to fluctuate.

6.73
Depersonalisation is often associated with a mood disorder.

6.74
Obsessive-compulsive disorder is commoner in women.

6.75
Compulsive acts are more closely associated with depression than obsessional thoughts.

6.76
In an acute stress reaction the affected individual is usually stunned for several hours.

6.77
Dissociative amnesia is typically anterograde.

6.78
Individuals with epilepsy usually share a number of characteristic personality traits.

6.79
Cruelty to animals as a child is associated with the development of personality disorders.

6.80
Characteristic features of anankastic personality include sensitivity to criticism.

6.81
Munchausen's syndrome is a delusional disorder.

6.82
Violent outbursts are typical of schizoid personality disorder.

6.83
Morbid jealousy is associated with personality disorder.

6.84
Personality disorder may be diagnosed secondary to brain disease.

6.85
Excessive self-importance is a typical feature of paranoid personality disorder.

6.86
Those with schizoid personality disorder have a heightened sensitivity to social norms.

6.87
The essential psychopathology in anorexia nervosa is regarded as a delusion.

6.88
Eating disorders are more commonly associated with a history of sexual rather than physical abuse.

6.89
Narcolepsy is associated with early-onset non-REM sleep.

6.90
The incidence of catatonic schizophrenia has decreased in developed countries due to the improved efficacy of neuroleptics.

6.91
All categories of schizophrenia in the ICD-10 require a minimum symptom duration of one month.

6.92
Atypicality is one of Bleuler's 'Four As' of schizophrenia.

6.93
Around 8% of subjects with psychosis have at least one Schneiderian first-rank symptom.

6.94
Concerning depression, circadian changes in mood are explained by changes in the secretion of melatonin.

6.95
There is a general lengthening of disease interval in bipolar disorder with increasing age.

6.96
Suicide rates are higher in bipolar illness than in recurrent depression.

6.97
Over time, those with bipolar illness generally experience more episodes of illness than those with unipolar disorder.

6.98
Pathological drunkenness classically presents with a swift impairment of consciousness.

6.99
Alcohol abuse is more commonly associated with depression than with mania.

6.100

Approximately 40% of the USA population have symptoms of caffeinism.

6.101

Visual hallucinations in schizophrenia are an example of a second-rank symptom.

6.102

There is a concordance rate of 10% for dissociative disorders among monozygotic twins.

Chapter 7: Psychiatric Assessment

7.1
The descriptions and guidelines given in the ICD-10 are based on psychiatric theory.

7.2
The ICD-10 recommends avoiding multiple diagnoses as much as possible.

7.3
Individuals with acute non-schizophrenic psychotic symptoms persisting over a month should nevertheless be classified as schizophrenic for the first three weeks.

7.4
The Beck Depression Inventory is a 21-point self-administered questionnaire.

7.5
In contrast to the ICD-10, the DSM-IV has not dispensed with the category of 'neurosis'.

7.6
When interviewing an individual who is confused, asking their date of birth is a good test of orientation.

7.7
Using closed questions is a good interview technique.

7.8
It is good practice to enquire about sexual history in the initial interview of someone presenting with depression.

7.9
Interpretation is a useful way of clarifying the history while interviewing a patient.

7.10
In the ICD-10, claustrophobia is categorised as a simple phobia.

7.11
In contrast to the ICD-10, the DSM-IV includes paraphrenia as a distinct diagnosis.

7.12
Like the DSM-IV, the ICD-10 is multi-axial.

7.13
Suicide mortality is higher in class V than in class I.

7.14
A brief depressive reaction should not persist beyond 2 weeks.

7.15
The Hamilton Rating Scale for depression cannot be accurately applied to individuals with a physical illness.

7.16
The majority of those who commit suicide do not have a psychiatric illness.

7.17
The Mini-Mental State Examination shows relatively poor inter-rater reliability.

7.18
Concerning the MMSE, the copying of intersecting polygons tests communication between the two cerebral hemispheres in a right-handed individual.

7.19
According to WHO guidelines, the combination of the CAGE questionnaire, MCV and GGT blood tests will pick up almost all cases of alcohol abuse.

7.20
The first question in the CAGE inventory is generally the most sensitive.

Chapter 8: Neurology/Medicine

8.1
Frontal lesions impair pursuit movements of the eyes.

8.2
Wartenberg's reflex is seen in frontal dementias.

8.3
Bell's palsy is the commonest cranial nerve palsy seen in psychiatry.

8.4
In monocular diplopia the disturbance occurs when the normal eye is covered.

8.5
Intermittent incontinence is a recognised symptom of normal pressure hydrocephalus.

8.6
Adrenal hypoplasia is seen in severe depression.

8.7
In pregnancy, seizure frequency in those with epilepsy increases by up to 50%.

8.8
Argyll-Robertson pupils are reactive to light but not to accommodation.

8.9
In Alzheimer's disease, neurofibrillary tangles correlate more closely with disease severity than neuritic plaques.

8.10
Dysgeusia is seen in temporal lobe epilepsy.

8.11
Confabulation occurs in bilateral hippocampal destruction.

8.12
In Huntington's disease, there is loss of the beta-rhythm on an EEG.

8.13
Blockage of the left posterior cerebral artery may be associated with visual agnosia.

8.14
Non-dominant temporal lobe lesions do not impair the appreciation of music.

8.15
Papilloedema may be caused by cortical vein thrombosis.

8.16
Myotonic dystrophy may be associated with frontal baldness.

8.17
Subcortical dementias tend not to affect posture.

8.18
AIDS encephalitis does not generally affect gait.

8.19
The EEG is more sensitive for petit-mal epilepsy than for space-occupying lesions.

8.20
The suicide rate associated with depression in Parkinson's disease is relatively low.

Chapter 9: Psychotherapy

9.1
Defences employed in obsessive-compulsive disorder include projection and undoing.

9.2
Systemic therapy is associated with family therapists.

9.3
Structural family therapy is based on the concept of enmeshment.

9.4
Double-bind communication was first postulated by Minuchin.

9.5
The aim of supportive psychotherapy is sometimes said to be to maintain a patient through a difficult time.

9.6
In projective identification the subject projects aspects of him- or herself on to another and thus identifies with the other person.

9.7
Group therapy is helpful in social phobia.

9.8
Pairing is one of Yalom's therapeutic factors in group work.

9.9
Foulkes emphasised analysis of the group as a useful therapeutic technique.

9.10
Ego strength is poorly developed in obsessional personalities.

9.11
The concept of ego is used by Jungian analysts.

9.12
The depressive position in Kleinian theory is linked to manic defences.

9.13
Klein was one of the first theorists to describe object relations.

9.14
Nirvana is associated with Freud.

9.15
Integration and synthesis are basic ego functions described initially by Klein.

9.16
Goffman described the features of 'total institutions' which culminate in 'mortification'.

9.17
Discussion of counter-transference issues is less important in brief psychodynamic therapy.

9.18
Behavioural psychotherapies involve the strict application of learning theory.

9.19
The use of free association is important in cognitive therapy.

9.20
The term 'group therapy' was first used by Main.

Chapter 10:
Extended Matching Items

10.1 Theme: Neuropsychological tests

Options:

    A Bender's Visual Motor Gestalt

    B Halsted-Reitan Battery

    C Mini-Mental State Examination

    D Minnesota Multiphasic Personality Inventory

    E Raven's Progressive Matrices

    F Rorschach test

    G Shipley abstraction test

    H Stanford-Binet test

    I Thematic Apperception Test

    J Wechsler Adult Intelligence Scale

Lead in: Which of the above tests are described by the following?

1 Requires the completion of logical sequences. Tests abstract thinking.

2 Consists of 11 subsets: 5 performance and 6 verbal.

3 Involves the interpretation of 10 inkblots.

4 Intelligence scale used in testing children. Consists of 120 items.

10.2 Theme: Theorists

Options:

A Karl Abraham

B Alfred Adler

C Eric Berne

D Sigmund Freud

E Erich Fromm

F Carl Jung

G Melanie Klein

H Abraham Maslow

I Frederich Perls

J Donald Winnicott

Lead in: Which of the above are associated with the following?

1 Depressive position.

2 Good-enough mother.

3 Self-actualisation.

4 Gestalt therapy.

10.3   Theme: Defences

Options:

- A Denial
- B Displacement
- C Idealisation
- D Introjection
- E Projective identification
- F Reaction formation
- G Regression
- H Repression
- I Splitting
- J Sublimation

Lead in: Which of the above are described by the following?

1 An inability to integrate opposing aspects of personality.

2 The unconscious refusal to accept/acknowledge external reality.

3 Overestimation of an object's qualities.

4 The diversion of socially unacceptable instincts and drives into socially appropriate and creative activities.

10.4   Theme: Language and thought

Options:

A   Asyndesis

B   Concrete thinking

C   Fusion

D   Logoclonia

E   Paragrammatism

F   Prolixity

G   Schizophasia

H   Tangentiality

I   Verbigeration

J   *Vorbeireden*

Lead in: Which of the above are described by the following?

1   Interweaving of two differing elements of thought.

2   Flight of ideas.

3   Word salad.

4   Unable to entertain abstract thought.

10.5 Theme: Emotions

Options:

    A Alexithymia

    B Anhedonia

    C Anosodiaphoria

    D *Belle indifférence*

    E Dysphoria

    F Dysthymia

    G Emotional incontinence

    H Euthymia

    I Moria

    J *Verstimmung*

Lead in: Which of the above are described by the following?

1 Extreme lability of mood.

2 Inability to express one's emotions verbally.

3 Emotional indifference to disease.

4 Fatuous affect.

10.6 Theme: Delusions

Options:

    A Apophanous perception

    B Autochthonous delusion

    C Cotard's syndrome

    D De Clerambault's syndrome

    E Delusional mood

    F Ekbom's syndrome

    G Nihilistic delusion

    H Querulant delusion

    I Somatic passivity

    J Syndrome of Fregoli

Lead in: Which of the above are described by the following?

1 Delusional belief of negation and nothingness.

2 A form of delusional misidentification.

3 A primary delusion, one that appears fully formed and suddenly without any apparent connection with past or ongoing matters.

4 A delusion of control.

10.7   Theme: Perception

Options:

   A   Autoscopic hallucination

   B   Eidetic image

   C   Extracampine hallucination

   D   Functional hallucination

   E   *Gedankenlautwerden*

   F   Hypnogogic hallucination

   G   Lilliputian hallucination

   H   Pareidolia

   I   Reflex hallucination

   J   Running commentary

Lead in: Which of the above are described by the following?

1   Vivid, effortless illusion heightened in intensity with focusing of attention.

2   Recollection of a memory as an hallucination.

3   Hallucination perceived outside an individual's field of perception.

4   Visual hallucination of oneself.

10.8 Theme: Movement

Options:

    A Ambitendency

    B Athetosis

    C Catatonia

    D Chorea

    E Flexibilitas cerea

    F *Gegenhalten*

    G Mannerism

    H *Mitmachen*

    I Obstruction

    J Stereotypy

Lead in: Which of the above are described by the following?

1 Serpentine, writhing movements involving extremities and facial muscles.

2 Repetitive, spontaneous, complex movements that were once purposeful.

3 Abrupt, jerking movements involving varying groups of muscles.

4 Individual is unable to complete an action, repeatedly starting and stopping.

10.9 Theme: Agnosia

Options:

A Agraphagnosia

B Anosognosia

C Anosodiaphoria

D Astereognosia

E Autotopagnosia

F Colour agnosia

G Hemisomatagnosia

H Finger agnosia

I Prosopagnosia

J Simultagnosia

Lead in: Which of the above are described by the following?

1 Unable to recognise faces.

2 Inability to recognise the form or shape of objects by palpation.

3 Forms part of Gerstmann's syndrome.

4 Tactile agnosia.

10.10 Theme: Aphasias

Options:

    A Anomic aphasia

    B Aprosody

    C Basal ganglia aphasia

    D Broca's aphasia

    E Conduction aphasia

    F Global aphasia

    G Thalamic aphasia

    H Transcortical aphasia

    I Wernicke's aphasia

Lead in: Which of the above are most likely to be produced by a lesion to the following?

1 Localised dominant angular gyrus damage.

2 Supramarginal gyrus containing arcuate fasciculus.

3 Inferior frontal gyrus. Motor speech area.

4 Auditory association cortex – superior temporal gyrus.

10.11 Theme: Memory

Options:

 A Declarative-episodic memory

 B Declarative-semantic memory

 C Encoding

 D Multi-store model

 E Procedural memory

 F Registration

 G Retroactive inhibition

 H Sensory memory

 I Short-term memory

 J Working memory

Lead in: Which of the above are described by the following?

1 Knowing 'how' to do things.

2 Large capacity; memories are unprocessed and last less than half a second

3 Also known as primary memory.

4 Also referred to as autobiographical memory.

10.12 Theme: Validity

Options:

A   Concurrent validity

B   Construct validity

C   Content validity

D   Convergent validity

E   Criterion validity

F   Cross validity

G   Divergent validity

H   Face validity

I   Incremental validity

J   Predictive validity

Lead in: Which of the above are described by the following?

1   Whether the intended characteristic appears to be measured.

2   The extent to which all aspects of the subject matter are assessed.

3   The extent to which a new measure approximates to true validity offering additional benefit and improving on other measures.

4   The degree to which a measure discriminates that being assessed from unrelated measures.

10.13 Theme: Personality

Options:

    A Bannister

    B Cattel

    C Cloninger

    D Erikson

    E Eysenck

    F Kelly

    G Kretschmer

    H Rogers

    I Rorschach

    J Sheldon

Lead in: Which of the above are most closely associated with the following?

1 The 'ideal self' which everyone tries to cultivate.

2 Described neuroticism, extroversion and introversion.

3 Derived 16 first-order personality factors.

4 Described athletic, asthenic and pyknic body-build.

10.14 Theme: Sexual development

Options:

    A Gender identity

    B Gender role

    C Sex typing

    D Sexual conflict

    E Sexual desire

    F Sexual drive

    G Sexual identity

    H Sexuality

    I   Sexual maturity

    J Sexual orientation

Lead in: Which of the above best describes the following?

1 Sexual partner preference.

2 The primary need for sexual gratification.

3 Behaviours that correspond to gender.

4 Differential treatment of different-sex children.

10.15 Theme: Antidepressants

Options:

- A Amitriptyline
- B Fluoxetine
- C Imipramine
- D Mianserin
- E Mirtazapine
- F Moclobemide
- G Phenelzine
- H Reboxetine
- I Sertraline
- J Venlafaxine

Lead in: Which of the above are described below?

1 A selective noradrenaline reuptake inhibitor.

2 A dual-action antidepressant that is an antagonist at serotonergic receptors.

3 A monoamine oxidase-B inhibitor.

4 A sedative tetracyclic.

10.16 Theme: Genetic disorders

Options:

    A Cri-du-chat syndrome

    B Fragile X syndrome

    C Hurler's disease

    D Kleinfelter's syndome

    E Lesch–Nyhan's syndrome

    F Neurofibromatosis

    G Phenylketonuria

    H Rett's disorder

    I Turner's syndrome

    J Tuberose sclerosis

Lead in: Which of the above disorders feature the following stigmata?

1 Ovarian dysgenesis, webbed neck, atrial septal defects, normal intelligence, cubitus vagus, Hashimoto's thyroiditis.

2 Corneal clouding, kyphosis, hepatosplenomeagly, bone thickening, enlarged head size.

3 Café-au-lait patches, axillary freckling.

4 Butterfly rash, shagreen patches, epilepsy.

10.17 Theme: Genetic disorders

Options:

    A Down's syndrome

    B Huntington's disease

    C Kleinfelter's syndrome

    D Lesch-Nyhan's syndrome

    E Myotonic dystrophy

    F Prader-Willi's syndrome

    G Schizophrenia

    H Tay-Sachs' disease

    I Turner's syndrome

    J Wilms' tumour

Lead in: Which of the above are described by the following?

1 Metabolic autosomal-recessive disorder.

2 Involves partial deletion of autosomal chromosome and results in small hands, feet and height.

3 Individual has an extra X-chromosome but is phenotypically a male.

4 Affected individual has hyperuricaemia, choreoathetosis and seizures.

10.18 Theme: Neuroendocrinology

Options:

    A Arginine vasopressin

    B Cholecystokinin

    C Cortisol

    D Enkephalin

    E Growth hormone

    F Prolactin

    G Pro-opio-melanocortin

    H Somatostatin

    I TSH

    J Vasoactive intestinal polypeptide

Lead in: Which of the above are described by the following?

1 Anterior pituitary release is inhibited by dopamine.

2 Pentapeptides are found both centrally and peripherally.

3 Pituitary release is inhibited by somatostatin and indirectly stimulated by noradrenaline and acetylcholine.

4 Plasma levels are raised in depression and diminished in chronic fatigue syndrome.

10.19 Theme: Neurochemistry

Options:

   A Acetylcholine

   B Adrenaline

   C Dopamine

   D Glutamate

   E Glycine

   F GABA

   G Histamine

   H Myo-inositol

   I Noradrenaline

   J Serotonin

Lead in: Which of the above are described by the following?

1 Excitatory amino acid.

2 Synthesised from histidine.

3 Inhibitory amino acid synthesised from serine.

4 Found in high concentrations in central raphe nuclei and synthesised from tryptophan.

10.20 Theme: Neuropathology

Options:

A   Alzheimer's disease

B   Binswanger's disease

C   Creutzfeldt–Jakob disease

D   Hellervorden–Spatz disease

E   Huntington's disease

F   Multi-infarct dementia

G   Pick's disease

H   Progressive supranuclear palsy

I   Punch-drunk syndrome

J   Wilson's disease

Lead in: Which of the above are described by the following?

1   Has characteristic 'knife-blade' brownish gyri with swollen cortical pyramidal cells.

2   Disorder of copper-carrying globulin.

3   Prion disease.

4   Has excessive trinucleotide repeats on short arm of chromosome 4.

10.21 Theme: Psychiatric diagnoses

Options:

A Delusional disorder

B Paranoid personality disorder

C Delirium

D Schizophrenia

E Postpartum blues

F Major depression

G Schizoid personality disorder

H Mania

I Anorexia nervosa

J Dementia

Lead in: Select the option most closely associated with the following:

1 Thought broadcasting and bizarre delusions of being controlled.

2 Grandiose delusions with expansive or irritable mood.

3 Somatic delusions and delusions of guilt with psychomotor retardation.

4 Mistrust and suspiciousness of people.

10.22 Theme: Affective Disorders

Options:

- A Cyclothymia
- B Double depression
- C Major depression
- D Bipolar I Disorder
- E Bipolar II Disorder
- F Dysthymia
- G Psychotic depression
- H Resistant Depression
- I Schizoaffective disorder
- J Combined depression

Lead in: Select the option best defined by the following:

1 Recurrent hypomanic episodes interspersed by periods of depression.

2 Combination of major depressive episodes and dysthymia.

3 Occurrence of recurrent brief depression together with episodes of major depression.

4 Delusions of guilt and nihilism with inanition and diminished self-care.

10.23 Theme: Anxiety Disorders

Options:

A Obsessive compulsive disorder

B Generalised anxiety disorder

C Social phobia

D Panic disorder

E Specific phobia

F Agoraphobia

G Post-traumatic stress disorder

H Body dysmorphic disorder

I Globus hystericus

J Tourette's syndrome

Lead in: Select the option best defined by the following:

1 Sensation of 'lump in the throat' accompanied by episodic fear of choking and inability to breath.

2 A fear of heights.

3 Vocal and motor tics.

4 'Railway spine'.

10.24 Theme: Antipsychotics

Options:

    A Haloperiodol

    B Olanzapine

    C Chlorpromazine

    D Risperidone

    E Quetiapine

    F Zuclopenthixol

    G Clozapine

    H Amisulpiride

    I Trifluoperazine

    J Droperidol

Lead in: Select the option most closely associated with the following:

1 Weight gain and potentially fatal agranulocytosis.

2 Neutropenia but not agranulocytosis. Rhinitis, ocular disturbances and priapism.

3 Often administered intramuscularly and as a depot injection.

4 Typical antipsychotic with a piperazine side-chain.

10.25 Theme: Culture-bound and other psychiatric syndromes

Options:

A Pseudologia fantastica

B Neurasthenia

C Amok

D Koro

E Chronic fatigue syndrome

F Cotard's syndrome

G Piblokto

H Paraphrenia

I Wihtigo

J Briquet's syndrome

Lead in: Select the option best described by the following:

1 A sudden unprovoked outburst of wild rage in which the individual attacks indiscriminately.

2 Attacks usually involving Eskimos during which a person tears off their clothing and screams.

3 Characterised by delusion that penis is shrinking and may disappear abdominally.

4 Affected person believes they may be transformed into a human flesh-eating monster.

Answers to Chapter 1: Basic Psychology

1.1

True: This is delayed conditioning. The least effective method is trace conditioning, in which the conditioned stimulus ends before the unconditioned stimulus begins.

1.2

False: Acquisition stage.

1.3

False: In contingency (or continuous) reinforcement, a behaviour is quickly acquired and the response rate is at its maximum. In partial reinforcement, where a reward is only occasionally given, variable reinforcement is more effective than a fixed schedule.

1.4

True: This theory holds that opposing emotions cannot exist simultaneously and is used as the basis for systematic desensitisation.

1.5

False: This is punishment. Negative reinforcement involves the removal of an aversive stimulus in response to a wanted behaviour.

1.6

True: The experimenters induced a fear of white rats into 'little Albert' (an 11-month-old boy) and then generalised the fear, initially to white rabbits and later to any furry object.

1.7

False: The conditioned response. For example, at the start of Pavlov's experiment salivation is an unconditioned response (to food) but later becomes the conditioned response (to the bell).

1.8
True: Operant conditioning is also known as instrumental learning.

1.9
True: This is observational learning.

1.10
False: The main components are continuity, closure, proximity, similarity and simplicity.

1.11
False: Object constancy refers to the ability to perceive an object as being the same despite changes in lighting, distance and orientation. Object permanence refers to the insight acquired in infancy that objects continue to exist when out of sight.

1.12
True: For example, on viewing a musical manuscript a layperson 'sees' a mass of unintelligible symbols whereas a musician would 'perceive' the same manuscript very differently.

1.13
False: He focused more on the attributes of the person being observed.

1.14
True: The ego and superego span the conscious and unconscious to varying degrees.

1.15
True: Too much or too little arousal is detrimental to performance.

1.16
True: Chaining involves breaking the behaviour into manageable parts. Shaping is an iterative technique that involves successively improved approximations.

1.17
False: It is a cognitive model.

1.18
True: Seligman's experiments involved dogs.

1.19
True: It is actually very difficult, if not impossible, to break a visual or auditory perception into its constituent parts.

1.20
True: First postulated by Weber, Fechner subsequently stated the relationship mathematically. Although in this particular form the law very often breaks down (ie the mathematical relationship does not always hold), the principle is nevertheless valid.

Answers to Chapter 2: Neuropsychological Assessment

2.1
True: As are the Rorschach inkblot, thematic apperception and 'complete a sentence' tests.

2.2
True: Although not strictly a measure of intelligence, the NART (which involves lists of words with unusual pronunciations) has been shown to have a positive association with IQ.

2.3
False: The leniency error is the tendency to avoid extreme responses.

2.4
False: It is important in the Cannon–Bard theory. The James–Lange theory states that emotions are secondary to physiological states.

2.5
True: This is because cognitive dissonance is unpleasant and individuals are therefore motivated to avoid it or reduce it to a tolerable equilibrium.

2.6
False: This is ideographic research. Nomothetic research pools information from population studies.

2.7
True: There are seven tiers in all, with basic physical needs at the bottom and self-actualisation at the peak.

2.8
False: This is reliability. Validity is a measure of the extent to which a test measures what it purports to measure.

2.9
False: Such a factor is believed to exist, though there is no agreed single test for it. It is usually designated by the letter g.

2.10
False: This term was coined by Sheldon. Both formulated categorical (as opposed to dimensional) theories of personality based on physical appearance. Most theorists no longer credit such theories.

2.11
True: The former is one of six verbal components and the latter one of five performance components.

2.12
True: Devised originally to assess brain damage, the HRNB provides a comprehensive overview of cognitive functioning. Ten individual tests are combined to give the overall Halstead Impairment Index, to which the WAIS and also the Minnesota Multiphasic Inventory are sometimes added.

2.13
True: Like Eysenck, Cattel took a dimensional approach to personality. Eysenck's work forms the basis of the Eysenck Personality Inventory.

2.14
False: They describe enhancements in short-term memory.

2.15
True: Declarative memory is further subdivided into semantic and episodic memory. Secondary memory is an alternative term for long-term memory.

2.16
True: It is used in assessing attitudes.

2.17
False: They are not regarded as naturally occurring.

2.18
False: Prosody, the intonation of speech, is usually localised to the right hemisphere.

2.19
True: Around 70–80% show it.

2.20
True: The olfactory bulbs are located in the phylogenetically older areas of the brain.

Answers to Chapter 3: Human Growth and Development

3.1
False: They require accommodation, which is the process of adjusting schemas or formulating new ones.

3.2
True: The depressive position is heralded by the child beginning to integrate good and bad aspects of the mother into a unified whole.

3.3
True: Much of his research was based on observations of his own children.

3.4
True: The infant relies on primitive defences (splitting, projective identification and introjection) in relating with its environment.

3.5
False: It spans ages 6 to 12 years, and ends with puberty.

3.6
False: It pertains principally to psychosexual development.

3.7
False: The oral (biting/sucking stages) and anal (sadistic/erotic stages) phases.

3.8
False: They show incorporation of objects. Ambivalence is seen in the anal stage.

3.9
False: It occurs from birth to 4 weeks.

3.10
True: These are differentiation, practising, rapprochement and object constancy.

3.11
True: The infant begins to realise that immediate gratification (initially through defaecation) creates conflict with the parents, thus realising that they cannot always do whatever they want whenever they want.

3.12
True: She wants to compensate for this loss by having a child by her father.

3.13
True: Introjection of parental attitudes forms the superego as part of this resolution.

3.14
True: During the first year, consistent love and satisfaction of needs will engender trust in the infant which will ultimately help to develop a healthy self-esteem (through notions of trusting oneself).

3.15
False: It occurs in adolescence and describes a stage between morality learned by the child and the ethics to be developed by adulthood.

3.16
True: The successful outcome is fulfilment.

3.17
True: The child gradually identifies more strongly with the same-sex parent and also begins to develop same-sex friendships.

3.18
True: This is observation under controlled conditions.

3.19
True: Others (such as Freud and Margaret Mahler) stopped with the onset of adulthood.

3.20
False: Attachment behaviour, most commonly associated with Bowlby, is most prominent from 6 months to 3 years of age.

3.21
True: Easy (40%), difficult (10%) and 'slow to warm up' (40%).

3.22
True: This is attachment with one individual (usually the main caregiver).

3.23
False: It appears at around 1 year.

3.24
True: Kohlberg's theory specifies six stages of moral development, arranged in three levels.

3.25
True: Typically those with personality disorders or antisocial traits.

3.26
True: The classic example is that of birds when hatching imprinting whatever they first see as their mother.

3.27
False: It is 0.2 metres.

3.28
True: The 6-metre measure is a convention, and would be equivalent to, say, 4:4 or 50:50 vision. What is important is the difference between the two numbers. So, for example, a person with 6:5 vision can read at 6 m what most people can only read from 5 m, ie they have better than average vision.

3.29
False: It is around half that.

3.30
False: It is slower to develop in children from large families.

3.31
False: It refers to the notion that certain fears appear to be more easily acquired, possibly due to an evolutionary genetic bias.

3.32
False: This is gender identity.

3.33
False: It is usually achieved by 5 years.

3.34
True: Breast enlargement.

3.35
False: It usually resolves within 6 to 12 months.

3.36
True: Denial, anger, bargaining, depression and acceptance.

3.37
False: It can be improved with practice and learning memory techniques. The problem is not usually one of retention but of recall.

3.38
False: Measured intelligence increases up until 16 years of age and then plateaus for approximately 10 years before entering into a gradual decline. Some individuals experience a 'terminal drop', which is a sharp decline in the final few years before death.

3.39
True: There is also an increase in sexual promiscuity and drug abuse.

3.40
False: They are likely to repeat the same patterns of behaviour.

Answers to Chapter 4: Psychopathology

4.1
True: This is thought echo. Other first-rank auditory hallucinations are commentary and third person.

4.2
True: It is the repetition of the last syllable of the last word.

4.3
True: It is part of the classification of thought disorder proposed by Cameron.

4.4
False: It is the subjective inability to describe how one is feeling.

4.5
True: For example, answering 'green' in response to 'What colour is the sky?'

4.6
False: This is *entgleiten*. *Entgleisen* is the displacement of one thought by another.

4.7
True: This is another term for a delusional perception.

4.8
False: This is Cotard's syndrome. Capgras is a syndrome of delusional misidentification.

4.9
False: Catatonia is a symptom of psychotic disorders characterised by abnormally increased or decreased (stupor) levels of activity.

4.10
True: This is thought echo. It is sometimes regarded as the simultaneous experience of thought and voice, whereas in *écho de la pensée* the thought precedes the voice.

4.11
True: Our only access to a person's thoughts is by their words and actions, so these terms are sometimes used interchangeably.

4.12
False: Not necessarily. For example, a man may (correctly) believe his wife is having an affair, but his only evidence is that the supermarket has reduced its prices.

4.13
False: There is no such term. Formal thought disorder pertains to the grammar, or 'form', of speech and language.

4.14
False: Thought echo is a characteristic type of auditory hallucination.

4.15
True: A stimulus in one sensory modality produces a percept in another, eg 'seeing' a piece of music as it is heard.

4.16
True: They are a common experience, eg misinterpreting a coat hanging on the door as being an intruder. They can be intensified with concentration.

4.17
False: It is characteristically incomprehensible, thus distinguishing this phenomenon from delusional misinterpretation.

4.18
True: Often on going to sleep or waking (hypnogogic and hypnopompic, respectively) or in a state of mental exhaustion.

4.19
False: They are pathognomic of psychosis.

4.20
True: Although they are not classified as delusions.

4.21
True.

4.22
True: The affected individual identifies strangers as people they know.

4.23
True: It is sometimes also described as the 'objective' (ie observed) mood.

4.24
False: Usually it refers to the apparent mismatch between a person's affect and the emotional context of what they are saying or the situation they are in.

4.25
True: This is different from an illusion in which both the stimulus and the percept are experienced as one (ie the percept is a distortion of the stimulus).

4.26
True: These are hallucinations of little people, seen in organic states such as alcohol withdrawal.

4.27
False: Rumination (an obsessional thought) is experienced as one's own, however unwanted or resisted it may be.

4.28
True: It can be thought of as being 'in between' normal thought and flight of ideas.

4.29
True: However, it is likely to return after a few months, possibly focusing on another area.

4.30
True: This is disorientation in a familiar environment due to an inability to remember the surroundings.

4.31
False: The experience must be attributed to an outside agency to qualify as passivity.

4.32
False: This is a term for the fatuous superficial moral sometimes seen in frontal lobe disorders.

4.33
True: According to Cameron, positive formal thought disorder includes over-inclusivity and flight of ideas. Negative formal thought disorder (alogia) includes concrete thinking.

4.34
True: The patient believes all or aspects of their surroundings have been exchanged for exact copies. A variant of Capgras Syndrome.

4.35
False: This is asyndesis, described by Cameron.

4.36
False: They have been described in temporal lobe epilepsy.

4.37
False: They are new words invented by the patient or a familiar word used in a novel way.

4.38
True: This is being careful about spending money.

4.39
False: In Couvade's syndrome the man believes he is pregnant. Pseudocyesis is a 'false pregnancy' experienced by women.

4.40
False: It has an overvalued idea, not a delusion, as its core psychopathology.

4.41
True: These are alternative terms for a primary delusion.

4.42
False: It is not seeing something that is there (ie no percept in the presence of a stimulus) in the absence of relevant organic pathology.

4.43
True: This is a term for delusional perception.

4.44
True: These are tactile hallucinations, and cocaine toxicity can give rise to the 'cocaine bug'.

4.45
False: These are hallucinations occurring outside the normal sensory range, and can, for example, involve hearing a voice in a different city.

4.46
False: It is the experience of seeing oneself and can be a pseudo- or a true hallucination.

4.47
False: They are never considered senseless, which helps distinguish them from an obsessional thought.

4.48
False: Partial delusions occur in a resolving psychosis and are less dominating than overvalued ideas.

4.49
True: Although it is not usual to do so, it is the perception of subjective movement (usually rotation) when none is taking place.

4.50
False: They are noises (eg knocking, running water). Complex hallucinations comprise voices and music.

4.51
True: This is 'delusional mood', where the patient has the vague but persistent sense that 'something', usually sinister (and always delusional), is happening or going to happen.

4.52
False: This is echolelia. Verbigeration is the repetition of fragmentary phrases.

4.53
False: They are current delusions relating to past events.

4.54
True: It is the opposite of *déjà vu*.

4.55
False: Seen in catatonia, parakinesia is a continuous irregular movement of the whole body. Mimicry of movement is termed echopraxia.

4.56
False: Seen in catatonia, this is an apparently motiveless resistance to any attempts by another to promote movement. It is also termed opposition or *Gegenhalten*.

4.57
False: Micropsia is a visual distortion caused by lesions to the eye or optic pathway in which objects appear smaller than they actually are. Macro- or megalopsia is the opposite, and the umbrella term is dysmegalopsia.

4.58
False: The experience of having thoughts removed is thought withdrawal. The essential component of thought broadcasting is of others being aware of, picking up on or participating in one's thoughts through some failure of confinement to one's head.

4.59
True: This is the sensation of crawling on the skin.

4.60
True: The patient believes they have a disease despite all evidence to the contrary. If they later turn out to have the disease they cannot be said to be delusional in this regard.

4.61
The content is usually genuine but it has been displaced in time or is not actually the personal experience of the individual concerned.

4.62
False: They address the person (eg 'you') or give commands.

4.63
False: This is the experience of seeing one's body from an external vantage point, and can occur, for example, in so-called 'near-death experiences' or sensory deprivation.

4.64
True. Derealisation occurs when the person experiences their environment as being somehow unreal and two-dimensional.

4.65
False: Seen in catatonia, this is where the patient lies with their head raised unsupported above the pillow or bed.

4.66
False: This is where a patient alternates movement between starting and retracting as if in a state of indecision, eg repeatedly offering their hand for shaking but then withdrawing it.

4.67
True: For example, believing oneself to have two left arms.

4.68
False: These describe opposite phenomena. Subjects experiencing phantom limb describe a continued (proprioceptive) awareness of a missing limb, whereas in hemisomatognosia the person experiences an intact limb as missing.

4.69
True: They are localised distortions, eg that one's ear is made of wood.

4.70
False: This is *mitmachen*. In *mitgehen*, the subject's limbs can be easily moved into any position, even if the subject is instructed to resist, despite intact neuromusculature.

4.71
True.

4.72
False: They involve the perception of water.

4.73
True: This helps to distinguish them from mannerisms, which may have (or have had) functional significance in certain situations, eg saluting.

4.74
True: There is, however, a concurrent impairment of consciousness.

4.75
True: The furrowed brow.

4.76
True: This is the experience of having two selves, or a 'double'.

4.77
False: It is a state of reduced range and degree of awareness in which the affected individual readily falls asleep.

4.78
True: Also known as 'snout spasm', this is where the rounded lips are thrust forward in an exaggerated whistling position.

4.79
False: This is catalepsy. Cataplexy is a temporary paralysis precipitated by emotion, and is a feature of narcolepsy.

4.80
False: Also known as 'photographic memory', the information is experienced as imagery and can therefore be suppressed at will.

Answers to Chapter 5: Psychopharmacology

5.1
True.

5.2
True: Fluoxetine is metabolised in the liver to norfluoxetine, which is then eliminated by the kidneys.

5.3
False: Two to three days. The metabolite, norfluoxetine, has a half-life of one week.

5.4
True: This can lead to hyperexcitability in the neonate.

5.5
True: This can cause neonatal goitre/hypothyroidism.

5.6
True.

5.7
False: It is more likely to cause flattened T-waves secondary to hypokalaemia.

5.8
False: It is absorbed as dimethyldiazepam, and is the only benzodiazepine not to be absorbed unchanged.

5.9
True.

5.10
True: By increasing lithium excretion.

5.11
True: Can be treated with beta-blockers. Lithium also exacerbates psoriasis.

5.12
False: α and θ activity is increased.

5.13
False: It increases their levels.

5.14
True: As can phenobarbitone, through folate deficiency.

5.15
True: An atypical antipsychotic, aripipazola also functions as a partial agonist at the 5-HT$_{1a}$ receptor and as an antagonist at the 5-H$_{T2}$ receptor.

5.16
True: It inhibits the suckling reflex.

5.17
False: It is a typical one.

5.18
True: Biperiden has a similar indication.

5.19
True: Due to decreased muscle blood flow.

5.20
False: It is potentiated.

5.21
False: Their effectiveness diminishes with time as the dementia progresses.

5.22
False: It is mainly by MAO-A.

5.23
True: By as much as ten times.

5.24
True.

5.25
True: Thioridazine had a similar side-effect profile, but was removed from the UK market largely due to its adverse cardiac effects.

5.26
True: Usually mild. However, due to the risk of underlying neutropaenia it is always important to exclude infection.

5.27
False: It is a sensitivity reaction (ie not dose-dependent).

5.28
True: As are diarrhoea and vomiting.

5.29
True: Patients may also complain of a mild emotional blunting.

5.30
True: Also a blackened tongue.

5.31
True: As can phenobarbitone.

5.32
False: It is the only MAOI with a significant sedative effect.

5.33
False: This combination of MAOI and TCA, respectively, is particularly dangerous.

5.34
False: It can cause a lowering of mood.

5.35
True: As are most mood stabilisers.

5.36
True: Smoking induces the cytochrome P450 CYP-1A2 and -2D6 enzymes which are important in the metabolism of planzapine.

5.37
True: Through their anti-adrenergic action.

5.38
True.

5.39
False: It may cause a syndrome of inappropriate antidiuretic hormone secretion (SIADH) which results in oliguria.

5.40
False: Carbamazepine interacts with MAOIs and enhances the inhibition of noradrenaline reuptake.

5.41
True: It is toxic to bone marrow.

5.42
False: It is the other way around.

5.43
True: Not common, but troublesome when it occurs.

5.44
True: An H_2-antagonist used in the treatment of peptic ulcers.

5.45
False: Hence they can be combined (with caution).

5.46
False: It is the other way around. These are anti-Parkinsonism drugs.

5.47
True: This is a centrally acting antihypertensive which has been found to be useful in Tourette's syndrome and attention deficit disorder.

5.48
True: Lofepramine is relatively non-sedating.

5.49
True: It is very sedating. Used as an adjunct in the treatment of resistant depression.

5.50
True: By MAO.

5.51
False: Although this is true of most drugs, alcohol and phenytoin metabolism has zero-order kinetics.

5.52
True: An idiosyncratic reaction.

5.53
True: Often more so.

5.54
True: It is prepared fish that is unsafe for those on an MAOI.

5.55
True: They also lower the seizure threshold.

5.56
True.

5.57
False: It is a precursor of 5-HT, not a neurotransmitter.

5.58
True: Used as an anti-emetic, domperidone can cause hyper prolacti-naemia and acute dystonic reaction.

5.59
True: Visual hallucinations are typical of acute organic states.

5.60
True.

5.61
True: Along with serotonin and noradrenaline.

5.62
False: AMPT inhibits tyrosine hydroxylase, thus lowering the synthesis of dopamine and noradrenaline, and precipitates a relapse in those recovered from depression who are not on maintenance medication. It thus has a similar effect to tryptophan depletion and little effect on healthy subjects.

5.63
False: It inhibits noradrenaline reuptake.

5.64
False: Usually four to five.

5.65
True: This interval is prolonged by most antipsychotic medications (especially the phenothiazenes) and patients on high doses or combination therapy should have regular ECG monitoring.

5.66
False: Usually within two to three hours.

5.67
False: 1 in 1000 births (0.1%), which is approximately a 20-fold increase over the general population.

5.68
True: This is true of phenytoin. Sodium valporate is associated with alopecia.

5.69
True.

5.70
False: An anti-epileptic that can be used as an adjunct in mania or bipolar disorder, topiramate is associated with anorexia and weight loss.

5.71
False: An anti-epileptic used to augment treatment in subjects with treatment-resistant partial seizures, gabapentin possesses a wide TI with a relatively benign side-effect profile.

5.72
False: It is generally seen within two weeks.

5.73
True: Typically from 25% of total sleep time to 10-15%.

5.74
False: A 5-HT$_{1A}$ partial agonist (antagonises release of 5-HT but agonises post-synaptic receptor) and classed as an anxiolytic, buspirone has been shown to be effective in generalised anxiety disorder.

5.75
False: It has been reported in a number of untreated patients with schizophrenia.

5.76
False: It appears to affect both sexes equally, but elderly women may be more susceptible.

5.77
True: Amisulpiride has different dosing regimens for the treatment of positive and negative symptoms.

5.78
False: They may delay its onset, but the evidence is inconclusive.

5.79
True: Donepezil is an anticholinesterase used in the treatment of Alzheimer's disease; suxamethonium is a depolarising muscle relaxant used in anaesthesia.

5.80
False: Tricyclics, SSRIs and lithium have also all been implicated in NMS.

Answers to Chapter 6: Psychiatric disorders

6.1
True: They are swollen cortical pyramidal cells, also known as Pick cells.

6.2
True: Neurofibrillary tangles, plaques and septum pellucidum perforation are also seen (secondary to bruising).

6.3
True: There is a relatively greater loss of neuronal mass in the adjoining areas of the brain with MiD.

6.4
False: Presenelin-1. Presenelin-2 is located on chromosome 1.

6.5
False: The psychotic symptoms seen in Parkinson's disease are generally delusions and visual hallucinations.

6.6
False: It is anterograde amnesia (the inability to learn new memories).

6.7
False: Progressive dementia is a recognised complication of severe closed head injury.

6.8
True: This can sometimes help to differentiate between the two conditions.

6.9
False: Anger is seen in 60% of cases; mild euphoria is seen in 10%.

6.10
True: Organic dysfunction has a more adverse effect on performance scores than on the verbal scores.

6.11
True: This is the mimicry of movement and speech respectively.

6.12
False: This is seen in vascular dementia. In Alzheimer's disease there is diffuse Δ and τ-wave activity.

6.13
True: Life events are also four times more common preceding a depressive illness than in the general population.

6.14
False: It is more than trebled.

6.15
True: The syndrome may be delusional at an overhauled idea and involve tactile (on or under the skin) or somatic (deep) hallucinations.

6.16
False: It is around 1–1.5%.

6.17
False: It sometimes precedes the onset of a delusion as part of an emerging schizophrenic illness.

6.18
True: Conversely, a long insidious onset generally carries a worse prognosis.

6.19
True: The incidence increases to 30–50% in an open injury with brain laceration.

6.20
False: They occur less commonly. Psychotic episodes in people with epilepsy tend to be less severe and respond better to treatment.

6.21
False: It spans January to March. A negative bias is seen for July to September.

6.22
False: It is exacerbated. Hence treatment is often 'geographical' in the first instance (ie the couple are separated) rather than medical.

6.23
True: This is in contrast to chronic physical pains.

6.24
False: An association with HLA-DR1 has been widely reported.

6.25
False: The class distribution of the fathers of individuals with schizophrenia is not significantly different to that of the general population.

6.26
False: There is no increase in organic disorders, mental retardation or bipolar illness.

6.27
False: It is related to the level of distress and paranoia.

6.28
False: They have no prognostic significance.

6.29
False: They are absent in around 20% of cases.

6.30
False: It is around one third of that (ie 8%).

6.31
False.

6.32
True.

6.33
False: Bipolar disorders are equally common, but unipolar depressive disorders are twice as common in women.

6.34
False: However, it is true that there is an increased risk of unipolar illness in relatives of a subject with bipolar illness.

6.35
False: It is the other way around.

6.36
True: There is also a decrease in REM latency.

6.37
False: They are more typical of schizophrenia.

6.38
False: It is usually only resolved by the complete termination of the relationship.

6.39
True: Also, tearfulness is a recognised feature of mania.

6.40
True: As is overeating.

6.41
True: Patients recovered from mania states often report having felt sad despite appearances to the contrary.

6.42
True: This is an extreme form of emotional blunting.

6.43
True: It accounts for around a third of suicides following a head injury. Overall, neurotic disability is the commonest psychiatric sequel of head injury.

6.44
False: It is closer to 6%. The majority of depression is treated in primary care.

6.45
False: It is largely arbitrary, with 'severe disruption' and 'more or less complete disruption' (of work and social activities) cited in the ICD-10 as one of the main discriminators between the two diagnoses. DSM-IV introduces a duration criteria of four days.

6.46
False: This condition is characterised by brief (typically 2 to 3 days and certainly less than 2 weeks) depressive episodes that meet the criteria for a mild, moderate or severe depressive episode.

6.47
True: It is a distinct subtype.

6.48
True: The diagnosis requires four episodes.

6.49
True: The concordance rate in monozygote twins is 60–70% in bipolar illness and around 45–55% in recurrent depression.

6.50
True.

6.51
True.

6.52
False: It is a risk factor for depression.

6.53
False: The prevalence of neurotic disorders in the elderly is around 25–30%.

6.54
True: Due to the difference in ease of escape from the situation.

6.55
True: The perception of time is also often altered.

6.56
True: However, although denial is characteristic of fugue states it is not a defence used in depression.

6.57
True: However, it typically returns after a few months, perhaps focusing on another area of the body.

6.58
False: There is often an association.

6.59
True: In the mid-20s.

6.60
True: Affective and schizophrenic psychoses can also occur.

6.61
True.

6.62
False: It is the other way around.

6.63
True: This is the inability to stand or walk despite intact neuromusculature of the legs.

6.64
True: Usually depression or anxiety, or both.

6.65
True: It is regarded to be a neurotic disorder.

6.66
True: Although performed to reduce anxiety, obsessive rituals can exacerbate anxiety if not done exactly.

6.67
False: There is actually very little evidence.

6.68
False: Secondary amenorrhoea.

6.69
False: 75% of those with agoraphobia may suffer an attack.

6.70
False: The beliefs in hypochondriacal disorder are not of delusional fixity.

6.71
False: Although individuals may complain of feeling 'light-hearted', this does not usually involve a feeling of spinning.

6.72
False: This is in contrast with specific phobias, which are of relatively fixed intensity.

6.73
True: Usually depression or anxiety or both.

6.74
False: It is equally common in both sexes.

6.75
False: It is the other way around.

6.76
True: The symptoms are typically mixed and change frequently.

6.77
False: It is retrograde (ie memories before the event are affected).

6.78
False: The idea of an 'interictal personality disorder' or 'epileptic personality' is controversial.

6.79
True: Most commonly with antisocial personality disorder.

6.80
True: Also known as obsessional personality.

6.81
False: It is a personality disorder.

6.82
False: Social withdrawal and an emotional coldness are more typical features.

6.83
True: It typically features delusions or overvalued ideas of infidelity.

6.84
True: Termed 'organic personality disorder'.

6.85
True: Other features are a suspicious nature and a tendency to bear grudges.

6.86
False: They are relatively insensitive in this regard.

6.87
False: It is regarded as an overvalued idea.

6.88
True: Often stated, though some researchers dispute this bias.

6.89
False: Late-onset.

6.90
False: The reason for the decrease is not known.

6.91
False: Simple schizophrenia stipulates one year.

6.92
False: They are autism, ambivalence, affective incongruity and loosening of associations.

6.93
True: However, approximately 20% of those with chronic schizophrenia never manifest a first-rank symptom.

6.94
False: There is little evidence for this.

6.95
False: The episodes of illness usually become more frequent and of longer duration.

6.96
False: Up to 20% in anorexia and 10% in schizophrenia.

6.97
True: Studies have shown that in the long term (25 years or so) those with bipolar illness experience on average ten episodes of illness, whereas those with unipolar illness experience only five.

6.98
False: The usual presentation is senseless violence or abrupt-onset and out-of-character behaviour.

6.99
False: It is the other way around.

6.100
False: It is estimated at around 10%.

6.101
True: Schneider's second-rank symptoms include hallucinations other than those of the first rank, perplexity and mood disturbances.

6.102
False: There is no evidence for twin-pair concordance in conversion disorders.

Answers to Chapter 7:
Psychiatric Assessment

7.1
False: They carry no theoretical implications.

7.2
False: However, it does suggest assigning the diagnoses an order of precedence.

7.3
False: They can continue to be classified as acutely psychotic until the required duration for delusional disorder (three months) has been reached.

7.4
True: The Hamilton Depression Scale requires an assessor.

7.5
False: The DSM-IV contains no such major category.

7.6
False: This is more a test of memory.

7.7
True: Used appropriately (generally after starting with open questions), closed questions can be useful in obtaining specific information.

7.8
False.

7.9
False: Recapitulation (ie repeating back to the patient what you think they have said) is preferable.

7.10
True: Specific phobias (eg animal phobias) are sometimes termed simple phobias.

7.11
False: The DSM-IV does not retain the term.

7.12
True: The ICD-10 is laid out in a hierarchical manner.

7.13
True.

7.14
False: The cut-off is 4 weeks.

7.15
True: Many items are likely to be confounded.

7.16
False: The prevalence of mental illness in those who commit suicide has been said to be as high as 90%.

7.17
False: The reliability of the MMSE is one of its main strengths.

7.18
True: The visuo-spatial processing required takes place largely in the right hemisphere, and the left hemisphere controls the hand copying what is seen.

7.19
False: It will pick up around 75%.

7.20
True: Opinions differ as to the relative merits of the four components, but it is generally agreed that 'Have you ever thought you should cut down?' is the most useful in assessing potential alcohol abuse.

Answers to Chapter 8: Neurology/Medicine

8.1
False: Saccades are impaired. Occipital, parietal and brainstem lesions impair pursuit movements. Both can be impaired in schizophrenia.

8.2
True: This is a primitive reflex, also known as the palmo-mental reflex.

8.3
False: It is abducens palsy, affecting the lateral rectus muscle, causing the characteristic 'down and out' appearance of the eye.

8.4
True: It is caused by local lesions such as a retinal tear or lens dislocation.

8.5
True: It is also a symptom of dementia and ataxia.

8.6
False: Hypertrophy.

8.7
True: Most likely in the first two trimesters, the increase is related to sleep deprivation and changes in the plasma concentrations of anti-epileptic medication.

8.8
False: It is the other way around. Seen in neurosyphilis.

8.9
True.

8.10
True: This is impaired taste, and it can be experienced as part of an aura preceding a seizure.

8.11
False.

8.12
False: The α-rhythm is lost. There is also a general flattening throughout the frequency spectrum.

8.13
True: Also with dyslexia, hemianopia and diploplia.

8.14
False: There is reduced musical appreciation.

8.15
True: It is also caused by raised intracranial pressure.

8.16
True: Myotonic dystrophy can also cause irreversible intellectual decline, culminating in an 'obstructive' personality.

8.17
False: They generally do affect it (eg Parkinson's disease, Huntington's disease).

8.18
False: It may also cause a head and neck tremor.

8.19
False: It is abnormal in around 75% of patients with an abscess, subdural haemorrhage, metastases or glioblastoma multiforme.

8.20
True.

Answers to Chapter 9: Psychotherapy

9.1
False: They are undoing, reaction formation and isolation.

9.2
True: It originated in Milan.

9.3
False: This is family systems theory.

9.4
False: It was postulated by Bateson. Minuchin is associated with enmeshment, and therefore with structural family therapy.

9.5
True: Psychodynamic therapy aims to effect change.

9.6
True: A primitive defence, associated most strongly with Klein.

9.7
True.

9.8
False: It is one of three 'basic assumptions' described by Bion. Yalom described 12 main factors in all.

9.9
False: Bion and Ezriel are associated with this.

9.10
False: It is highly developed, but poorly developed in obsessive-compulsive disorder.

9.11
True.

9.12
True.

9.13
True: Though not generally considered to be an object relations theorist.

9.14
True: In *The Project*, Freud described this as a tendency to decrease excitation to a minimum.

9.15
True.

9.16
True: He described mechanisms within a closed institution (eg prison) by which an individual becomes institutionalised and anonymous.

9.17
False: Early discussion is important.

9.18
True: For example, using systematic desensitisation in the treatment of phobia disorders.

9.19
False: This is an early method of psychoanalysis employed by Freud.

9.20
False: It was first used by Moreno. Main's name is associated with therapeutic communities.

Answers to Chapter 10:
Extended Matching Items

10.1

1:G
2:J
3:F
4:H

10.2

1:G   Also associated with paranoid–schizoid position.
2:J   Studied mother–baby relationship.
3:H   Maslow's pyramid.
4:G

10.3

1:I
2:A
3:C
4:J

10.4

1:C   *Verschmelzung*. Proposed by Schneider.
2:F   Train of thought eventually returns to original track.
3:G
4:B

10.5

1:G
2:A
3:C
4:I   *Witzelsucht*: apathy and silliness combined with general indifference.

10.6

1:G   Occurs in Cotard's syndrome.
2:J
3:B
4:I

10.7

1:H
2:B   Common among children.
3:C
4:A   *Doppelgänger.*

10.8

1:B   Absent in sleep.
2:G   Contrast with stereotypy (not goal-directed, and are socially unacceptable).
3:D
4:A

10.9

1:I   Mirror sign in Alzheimer's disease.
2:D
3:H   Other components include agraphia, right–left disorientation, acalculia, alexia.
4:A   Unable to identify figures (numbers/letters) drawn on palm. Also called agraphaesthesia.

10.10

1:A
2:E
3:D   Expressive aphasia. BA 44 and 45.
4:I   Receptive aphasia. BA 22 and 42.

10.11

1:E
2:H
3:I   Allows conscious processing of information. Fades in 20–30 seconds.
4:A   Long-term memory for events and places.

10.12

1:H
2:C
3:I
4:G

10.13

1 H   Rogers's self-theory. Every person strives for fulfilment.
2:E   Also psychoticism.
3:B   Further analysed these to develop three dimensions: intelligence, sociability and anxiety.
4:G   As did Sheldon. However, he used the terms meso-, ecto- and endo-morphy.

10.14

1:J   For example, heterosexual, homosexual and bisexual.
2:F
3:B   Masculine, feminine, etc.
4:C   Impacts upon gender identity and gender role.

10.15

1:H   Alpha-2 receptor antagonist.
2:E H_1, alpha$_2$, $5HT_2$ and $5HT_3$ receptor antagonist.
3:G   Moclobemide acts only on MAO-A.
4:D   Main adverse effect is that of sedation.

10.16

1:I   XO, occurs in 1 in 2500 female births.
2:C   Gargoylism.
3:F
4:J   Adenoma sebaceum.

10.17

1:H   Defect of hexosaminidase A.
2:F   Also small testicles.
3:C   XXY.
4:D   Deficiency of hypoxanthine phosphoribosyl transferase in purine metabolism.

10.18
1:F
2:D
3:E
4:C

10.19
1:D
2:G
3:E
4:J

10.20
1:G   Balloon cells.
2:J   Caeruloplasmin deficiency.
3:C
4:E   Autosomal dominant, occurs in 1 in 20,000 cases.

10.21
1:D   Individual believes that their thoughts are shared with others by virtue of them being somehow broadcast eg by telepathy. Characteristic of schizophrenia.
2:H   Individual is often irritable, elated or expansive in mood with pressure of speech and racing thoughts that can be expressed as clang associations and punning.
3:F   Psychomotor retardation is a core feature of melancholia in which the patient often feels excessive guilt.
4:B   This is a longstanding feature of paranoid personality disorder.

10.22
1:E   In bipolar I disorder the individual must have experienced at least one manic episode. Bipolar II is more common than Bipolar I disorder.
2:B   A predominantly North American term that indicates the over-lapping of two patterns of illness.
3:J   A rarely used term that has little clinical salience.
4:G   Patient often has psychomotor retardation.

10.23

1:I

2:E

3 J

4:G   19th century description of patients affected by traumatic experiences – reflected the view that this had resulted in physical disruption of the nervous system.

10.24

1:G   Clozapine and olanzapine both cause significant weight gain. Clozapine causes reversible neutropenia (3%) and potentially fatal agranulocytosis (0.8%).

2:D   Also associated with rashes, insomnia, sexual dysfunction and sedation.

3:F   As zuclopenthixol acetate (Clopixol-acuphase) and zuclopenthixol decanoate depot.

4:I   Others include prochlorperazine and fluphenazine.

10.25

1:C   Malayan term used to describe such homicidal behaviour.

2:G   After attack person has no memory of the attack.

3:D   Affects males in Southeast Asia and China.

4:I   Occurs predominantly in North American native Indians.

Index